Child Abuse:
A Quick Reference

Cynthia Feinen, RN, C
and
Winifred Coleman, RN, BSN

Vista Publishing, Inc.

Edited by Margaret Curry Ciocco, BSN, RN,C

Cover Design Thomas Taylor of Thomcatt Graphics

Original art work designed by Jason Feinen

Vista Publishing, Inc.
422 Morris Avenue Suite One
Long Branch, NJ 07740
(732) 229-6500
www.vistapubl.com

This publication has been designed to provide basic information regarding the subject of child abuse. The authors do not hold any claim that this information is the only information required by the professional in working with victims of child abuse. The authors strongly suggest and advise the reader to seek all references available in building a knowledge base in the subject area.

Printed and bound in the United States of America

First Edition

ISBN: 1-880254-52-2

Library of Congress Catalog Card Number: 97-62501

USA Price $24.95
Canada Price $29.95

"When I finished reading this manuscript, I felt mentally exhausted. The text is well written and easy to read. It's the subject matter. However, in today's world this is a much needed reference source.

As an educator, I was impressed with the ease with which I was able to read the material. I wasn't bogged down by incomprehensible medical terms, and those that were included were plainly defined. An extra bonus to the manuscript was the bibliography of reference sources.

Ms. Feinen and Ms. Coleman did an excellent job of presenting this information on child abuse. Hopefully education, medical people and anyone in the profession of caring for children will include this as an important purchase for their reading shelf."

Mary McCaffery, BA
Elementary Education
K-8

Dedication

For all the children who have shed tears unnecessarily,
        cowered in fear,
                kept secrets because they were afraid to tell
                and ...
                        died nameless.

Special Thanks

To Carolyn Zagury for her unwavering support, positive reinforcement and encouragement during the writing of this book.

Meet The Authors

Authors Cynthia Feinen and Winifred Coleman are Registered Nurses with extensive experience in working with victims of child abuse. They have worked with families to identify and prevent potential child abuse situations and have developed and presented numerous educational programs on child abuse and prevention for community groups, professionals and health care providers. Both maintain multiple professional affiliations.

Cynthia is a graduate of Ann May School of Nursing in Neptune, New Jersey and maintains her certification in pediatrics. Her background includes general pediatrics, pediatric intensive care, pediatric emergency and trauma, community health nursing, nurse manager of a residential Pediatric Aids Program and CPR instructor. She is also trained death investigator.

Through her work with families and abused children, Cynthia has developed assessment tools and educational programs to assist medical, nursing and social work professionals to better identify and assist victims of child abuse.

Winifred received her nursing diploma from the Bridgeport Hospital School of Nursing in Bridgeport, Connecticut and her BSN from Monmouth University, West Long Branch, New Jersey. Her background includes medical surgical nursing, burn unit nursing, intensive care, adult and pediatric mental health (both inpatient and outpatient care), intensive care pediatric psychiatric unit, mental health screening, research, high tech pediatric home care and general pediatrics. She has held numerous management positions including Director of a Mental Health Division for Managed Care and Director of Nursing of a Substance Abuse Rehabilitation Center.

Winifred is currently working to develop critical pathways which will be utilized by health care providers, case managers and professionals in the field of child protection.

Forward

As a practicing Pediatrician for 32 years, I continue to be amazed by the growing number of child abuse cases each year. The *"war" on child abuse* requires continual education and diligent observation by all of those who work with children. The signs and symptoms of child abuse are at times blatant and, at times very subtle.

In my experience, I have seen a great number of children that have been both abused and neglected. This book is extensive, yet an easy to read reference that will assist the practitioner in identifying child abuse.

Everyone, from parents to pediatricians should have this book. All too often we hear the words, "I do not want to get involved", words that ignore the potential risk to the child. At times, the physician, nurse and teacher are not able to identify the signs and symptoms of abuse due to the lack of sufficient education and training in the field.

Ms. Feinen and Ms. Coleman have extensive and varied experience in the fields of nursing, mental health and child abuse. They have done an exceptional job in bringing their experience and expertise together through the writing of this book.

The war on child abuse is a fight everyone must become a part of. **Child Abuse: A Quick Reference** is a must read for everyone who cares for and cherishes our children.

Joseph C. Bogdan, MD

Author Note: Distinguished in the field of pediatrics, Dr. Bogdan has extensive experience in child in child abuse detection and prevention including:
Director of Pediatrics, Jersey Shore Medical Center
Director, Child Abuse Diagnostic Center, Jersey Shore Medical Center
Member, Governor's Task Force on Child Abuse
Member, Monmouth County Prosecutor's Child Abuse Task Force

TABLE OF CONTENTS

TABLE OF CONTENTS

TABLE OF CONTENTS

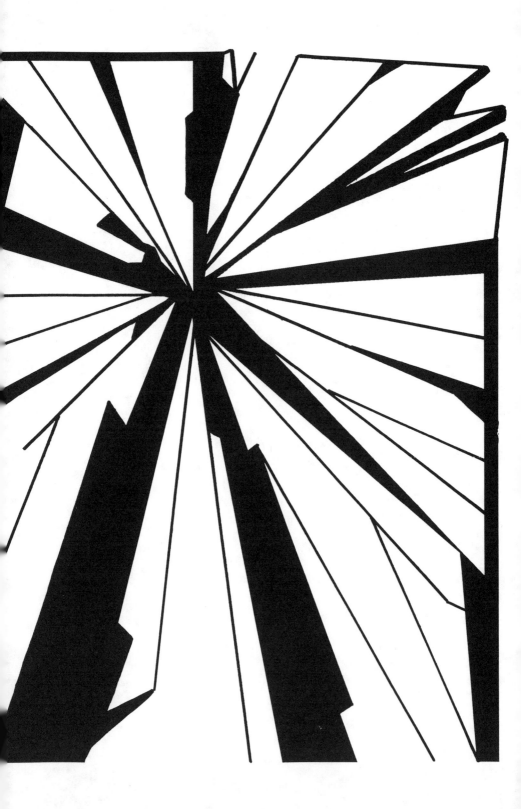

Introduction

The primary goal of this book is to provide the reader with the basic information needed to identify and report child abuse, thus assisting in the prevention and treatment of child abuse.

The number of victims of child abuse is increasing. The most recent statistics state that there are over 4.2 million child abuse referrals made each year. This book has been written to be used as a quick reference for those who are working with children in order to identify all aspects of child abuse. This book should not be considered as a replacement for a comprehensive knowledge of child abuse.

This book will assist the professional in identifying the indicators, physical findings and psychosocial aspects of the abused child and his/her family. It will also cover information on reporting, legal considerations and resources available.

The format of the text is designed to give general information regarding the abuser and the victim. The format is user friendly and utilizes tables, brief descriptions and diagrams.

In an attempt to maintain the quick reference text, prevention and treatment have been limited to information on reporting child abuse and resources available.

CHAPTER ONE

PSYCHOSOCIAL ASSESSMENT

The psychosocial assessment is the initial aspect of the investigation. A good psychosocial assessment will aide in determining the direction to pursue the investigation and prepare for the forensic interview.

The following information should be included in the initial psychosocial assessment:

Demographic Data of the Victim
Name
Address
Date
D.O.B
Statement of problem/description of the injury

Family History of the Victim

Family Composition
All significant individuals
Age of the parents or primary care givers
Current parties living at same address
Relationships between family members
With whom does the victim feel closest
Family supports systems
History of Police involvement

General Health of the Family Members
History of mental illness, depression
History of drug or alcohol use
History of domestic violence
History of chronic medical condition

Family Support Network
> Who to contact in case of an emergency
> Person the victim feels most comfortable with when in crisis

Financial Situation of the Victims Household
> Source of income
> Medical insurance

Medical History of the Victim

Birth History
> Pregnancy - number of
> Labor - how many hours
> Delivery - vaginal or cesarean

Developmental Milestones
> Delayed or on target

History of Hospitalizations

History of Past Accidents or Injuries

Identify Primary Care Physician
> Last medical exam (when and where)
> Seeks treatment for acute illnesses or preventative care

Current Family Stresses
> Losses - death, divorce
> Financial difficulties
> Inadequate housing and clothing
> Limited food availability
> Other stresses identified

Mental state
> Judgment
> Mood
> Insight into problem
> Thought processes
> Orientation

Following this psychosocial assessment, the investigation proceeds to the forensic interview. There have been numerous articles written about the forensic interview. The legal system is intricately involved in this process. The following is a sample of the information needed:

✓ Time and date of injury

✓ Events leading to injury

✓ Cause of injury reported by whom

✓ The identity of the primary care giver

✓ Location of incident

✓ Location of the care giver

✓ Names of witnesses to the incident

✓ Amount of time that had elapsed prior to medical care being sought

✓ Was hospitalization required

✓ Who brought victim to hospital

✓ If medical care was not provided, why not

✓ Assess the appropriateness of the response by the parents or evaluate the consistency of history to the injury

Details on how, where, who and when this interview takes place will depend upon the policies and procedures of individual organizations. Familiarity with these policies and procedures and all state regulations, guidelines and laws regarding child abuse are essential.

PROFILE OF AN ABUSER

The profile of an abuser can be described by several specific qualities which include external factors, personality features of the abuser, specific history of events and stress factors. The characteristics of the child may also contribute to the abuse. Any one of these situations may "trigger" an abusive situation. Any combination of factors should be considered a high risk situation.

The *external factors* are those situations in which high risk factors can precipitate an abusive situation. These situations include, but are not limited to:

⇨ Teen parent

⇨ Substance abusing parent or caretaker

⇨ Depressed caretaker- chronic or acute illness

⇨ Single parent home with an unstable home life

⇨ Poorly organized lifestyle-distorted priorities in family life

⇨ Poor father figure who is unwilling or unable to assert a controlling influence on the family

⇨ Chronic impoverishment

⇨ Chronic medical problems of the abuser

Certain *personality characteristics* of an abuser have also been identified when defining the anatomy of an abuser and can be identified by the professional during the interview and assessment process. They may include, but are not limited to, the following:

⇨ Inappropriate behavioral expectations for the age of the child

⇨ A need to be in control

⇨ Low self-esteem

⇨ Poor self understanding

⇨ Poor impulse control

⇨ Social isolation

⇨ Emotional immaturity

⇨ Problems with anger management

⇨ Unrealistic expectations of what the child can provide emotionally to the abuser

⇨ Experiences outbursts of rage

⇨ Substance abuser

Specific *history events* that lead to patterns of abusive parenting or caregiving may include the following:

⇨ The abuser's childhood experience lacked affection or warmth

⇨ The environment was not conducive to the development of an adequate self esteem

⇨ History of violent or aggressive behavior

⇨ History of abuse as a child

⇨ History of domestic violence- witnessed or as a partner

⇨ Long term abusers are usually in their 30-40's

⇨ Majority of abusers are male but the incidence of female abusers is growing

⇨ History of intoxication (drug/alcohol) while caring for the child

⇨ Substance abusers who spend all their money, energy and time obtaining the abused substance.

Stress factors play an important role in abusive situations. Even the healthiest of families have difficulties during a crisis or stressful situation. The child is especially at risk if any of the following stress factors are present:

⇨ Sudden financial problems

⇨ Loss of a job

⇨ Loss of housing

⇨ Divorce or separation

⇨ Overcrowded housing

⇨ Change in the composition of family, such as a birth or additional extended family

Caring for any child can be challenging even when the situation is ideal. A difficult child can test any caregiver's parenting skills. For this reason the child that has special needs may be at higher risk for being abused. Characteristics of these children may be, but not limited to the following:

⇨ Those with behavioral problems

⇨ The child with Attention Deficit Hyperactive Disorder (ADHD)

⇨ A premature infant

⇨ An infant with colic

⇨ A child under the age of five (due to their

developmental needs)

⇨ A chronically ill child

⇨ The drug exposed infant

⇨ The oppositional teen

⇨ Developmentally delayed

⇨ A child who is mismatched to parent's personality or similar to an adult that is disliked by the abuser

As you can see, the profile of the abuser is not one dimensional. The combination of factors at any given time produces the abusive event which creates the total picture. These factors must be understood in order to develop treatment and prevent future abuse.

CHAPTER TWO

REPORTING AND INTERVIEWING
OBLIGATIONS AND LEGAL CONSIDERATIONS

Everyone can help fight child abuse. The first step is reporting suspected abuse and neglect of the endangered child. Children are frequently too young and vulnerable to protect themselves or to report abuse. Helpless children can only be protected if there is a concerned individual that is able to "recognize" the danger or the risk of harm to the child.

Reporting child abuse is the first step in saving children from a future riddled with fear, pain and suffering. The method of reporting child abuse is frequently misunderstood. When considering if you should report a suspicious situation involving possible child abuse or neglect you must remember that the only factor you must consider is the *"risk of harm"*. If there is a risk of harm to the child due to the situation that you are aware of then that is enough to report. Failing to report a suspicion of abuse may expose a child to serious injury, harm or even death.

In the early 1960's, a model law was presented to The Children's Bureau to mandate that physicians report any child with "serious physical injuries, or injuries inflicted ... other than by accidental means." Within four years all fifty states enacted reporting laws that were patterned after the model law. Initially mandatory reporting laws were only directed at the physician and specifically for "serious injuries". The response of reports generated from this law encouraged most states to broaden the terms of child abuse reporting laws. The laws were broadened to incorporate all forms of "suspected" child abuse and/or neglect.

Many states now have expanded the laws regarding persons who are mandated to report child abuse. The initial laws centered around physicians seeing the actual injury. In an effort to prevent the child from injury, the laws were changed to encompass the suspicion of abuse. Thus the laws are focused on preventing the abuse. The change in the individuals that were mandated to report, focused on those people who saw the child more frequently than the physician. Those people that are mandated to report in all states are physicians, nurses, dentists, mental health professionals, social workers, teachers, school officials, day care or child care workers, and law enforcement personnel. If a person who is mandated to report does not, there are criminal and civil sanctions that may be pursued.

It is your moral obligation to report child abuse. In all states any person is allowed to report abuse or the suspicion of abuse. In twenty states, however, it is mandated that all citizens report abuse. In all states, anonymous reports are accepted and handled with the same priority as an identified report.

When investigating details and allegations it is much more efficient to interview the person who is calling. The caller may also have additional information regarding further leads in the investigation. The worker taking the call should attempt to convince the caller to identify themselves. The worker has no choice, however, but to accept the referral, if appropriate, even when anonymous.

In understanding what is reportable child abuse and neglect you must understand what the definitions are regarding reportable suspicions. The table of definitions on the following page is a guide to assist the professional in building a working knowledge of these important definitions. The Table is reprinted from *Recognizing Child Abuse: A Guide For The Concerned* by Douglas J. Besharov (1990, The Free Press).

In most states, a "child" is referred to as *anyone under the age of eighteen*. Most states feel that any child eighteen years of age or older is capable of protecting themselves. Many states have legislation that has a higher age cut off for special needs children (for example, those children who are mentally retarded, handicapped or disabled). In most states, these children have a cut off age of twenty years.

Deciding to report child abuse can be an agonizing decision. It is important to understand that the decision to report is based on good faith and necessary to prevent serious harm to a child. *Reporting a suspicion of abuse and preventing abuse may save a child's life!*

Table of Definitions

Physical abuse: physical assaults such as striking, kicking, biting, beating, throwing, burning or poisoning that caused or could have caused, serious physical injury to the child

Sexual abuse: vaginal, anal, or oral intercourse; vaginal or anal penetrations; and other forms of inappropriate touching or exhibitionism for sexual gratification

Sexual exploitation: use of a child in prostitution, pornography, or other sexually exploitative activities

Physical deprivation: failure to provide basic necessities such as food, clothing, hygiene, and shelter that caused, or over time would cause, serious physical injury, sickness or disability

Medical neglect: failure to provide the medical, dental, or psychiatric care needed to prevent or treat serious physical or psychological injuries of illnesses

Physical endangerment: reckless behavior toward a child such as leaving a young child alone or placing a child in a hazardous environment that caused or could have caused serious physical injury

Abandonment: leaving a child alone or in the care of another under circumstances that suggest and intentional abdication of parental responsibility

Emotional abuse: physical or emotional assaults such as torture and close confinement that caused or could have caused serious psychological injury

Emotional neglect (or developmental deprivation): failure to provide the emotional nurturing and physical and cognitive stimulation needed to prevent serious developmental deficits

Failure to treat a child's psychological problems: indifference to a child's severe emotional or behavioral problems or parental rejections or appropriate offers of help

Improper ethical guidance: grossly inappropriate parental conduct or lifestyles that pose a specific threat to a child's ethical development or behavior

Educational neglect: chronic failure to send a child to school

Reprinted with permission of The Free Press, a Division of Simon & Schuster from *Recognizing Child Abuse: A Guide for the Concerened* by Douglas J. Besharov. Copyright © 1990 by Douglas J. Besharov.

LEGAL LIABILITY

In almost all states it is a crime to fail to report suspected child abuse. Most states consider failure to report suspected child abuse as a misdemeanor. The punishment can be fines, a jail sentence or both. State laws regarding this subject, guide the prosecution in the case. There are many states in which the law is written that the mandated reporter willingly fails to report abuse when abuse is "observed". In other states it may be that the reporter "suspects" abuse. It is important to understand your state law regarding who is mandated to report and what exactly reporting means.

INTERVIEWING THE CHILD

Interviewing is a specific form of goal directed communication. The goal is to gather all the pertinent facts and the truth. If the child is able to talk it may be considered the most important part of child abuse investigation. Some of the guidelines and general rules for this interview are as follows.

Establishing the Setting

- ✓ Children will provide more accurate detail in an informal private setting

- ✓ The setting should be comfortable for the child

- ✓ There should be space to move around and explore

- ✓ Limit toys to decrease distraction

- ✓ The environment should be welcoming to the child

- ✓ It is not recommended to feed the child during the interview, however, the recommendation is to offer refreshment after the interview

- ✓ Choose a time when it is not likely that the child will be hungry or sleepy

- ✓ Assure privacy

- ✓ Parents or relatives that are closely involved with the child should not be present when the child is questioned about the abuse

- ✓ If the child is apprehensive, allow a support person to stay for the beginning of the interview

The Interviewer

- ✓ *Can* be of either sex as long as they are effective

- ✓ *Should* be sensitive and able to communicate with children

- ✓ *Should* introduce themselves to the child

- ✓ *Should* identify boundaries with the child, i.e. confidentiality (State that the child will not get in trouble for telling)

- ✓ *Should* request that the child be honest

- ✓ *Should* make the child feel comfortable

- ✓ *Should* initially ask easy questions

- ✓ *Should* share personal information such as your dogs name

- ✓ *Should* allow the child to have freedom to move about

- ✓ *Should* identify child's developmental level

- ✓ *Should* determine if child understands the difference between telling the truth and telling a lie

- ✓ *Should* speak at the child's language level

General Rules of Interviewing

✓ Ask open ended, simple, direct questions

✓ Ask "yes" or "no" questions which will test reliability

✓ Seek explanations of the "yes" or "no" answers

✓ Do not present questions in a accusatory way

✓ Never threaten or force a child to continue in an interview

✓ Validate the child's feelings

✓ Do not make promises you can't keep

✓ Define the interviewer's role and purpose of the interview

✓ Keep notes or record the interview, elicit the child's responses and explain the reason for the documentation

✓ Questions must be very concrete. Children do not think in the abstract

✓ End the interview on a positive note. Thank the child for being brave and doing well. Let them know how they can reach you if they remember anything else.

If at anytime during an interview with a child abuse is disclosed, a referral to the appropriate investigative team should be made immediately. The investigative team is specially trained, and is knowledgeable in effectively interviewing children, and pursuing the appropriate interventions of the legal system.

Protect Against Child Abuse

THINK ABUSE

1. *Recognize the danger to the child*

2. *Risk of harm*

3. *Decision to report is based on good faith*

4. *Report to child protective services*

CHAPTER THREE

INDICATORS OF ABUSE

Certain *signs, symptoms and behaviors may indicate abuse.* In this text, the most common indicators specific to each form of child maltreatment will be outlined.

PHYSICAL ABUSE

Physical abuse may be defined as *the non-accidental bodily injury or harm that a child experiences as a result of severe or persistent actions by the caregiver.*

These actions include, but are not limited to, the following:

Hitting
Punching
Beating
Kicking
Biting
Burning
Shoving
Shaking
Bruising
Choking
Suffocating

A number of these actions can be a result of excessive or inappropriate discipline. Actions used by the caretaker during discipline may not have been intended to severely injure the child.

PHYSICAL ABUSE INDICATORS

PHYSICAL INDICATORS OF THE VICTIM

Bruises and Marks

* Various stages of healing
* A visible pattern mark
* Defining shape
* Location such as torso, buttocks, face and mouth

Burns

* Oval or circular in shape
* Patterned
* Submersion

Fractures

* Multiple
* Various stages of healing
* Spiral
* Facial
* Skull

BEHAVIORAL INDICATORS OF THE VICTIM

* Withdrawal from adult contact
* Fearful of caretaker
* Aggressiveness
* Afraid to go home
* No stranger anxiety
* Low self esteem
* Denial
* Seeking approval

BEHAVIORAL INDICATORS OF THE CARETAKER

* Inconsistent history
* Multiple histories
* Blaming others for the injury
* Seeks care for recurrent injuries of the child
* Delay or refusal in seeking medical care
* Inappropriate response to the injury
* Developmentally inappropriate injuries

Protect Against Child Abuse

THINK ABUSE

1. *Bruises in various stages of healing*

2. *Bruises in locations such as the buttocks , face, torso and mouth*

3. *Afraid to go home*

4. *Inconsistent history from the caretaker*

5. *Developmentally inappropriate injuries*

EMOTIONAL ABUSE

Emotional abuse may be defined as *the lack or inability of the caretaker to meet the child's social, emotional, and intellectual developmental needs.*

PHYSICAL INDICATORS OF THE VICTIM

* Finger sucking
* Rocking
* Biting
* Sleep disorders
* Obsession
* Sadness
* Weight loss
* Destructive
* Solitary play
* Hypochondria

BEHAVIORAL INDICATORS OF THE VICTIM

* Attempted suicide
* Overly compliant, passive or withdrawn
* Overly aggressive, demanding or social
* Does poorly in school
* Bitter
* Resentful

BEHAVIORAL INDICATORS OF THE CARETAKER

* Ridicules
* Threatens child with beating or abandonment
* Exposes child to family violence
* Repetitious yelling
* Rejects the child
* Humiliates the child
* Uses child as scapegoat
* Lack of attention
* Conditional love
* Lack of bonding

SEXUAL ABUSE

Sexual abuse is defined as *the exploitation and/or sexual activity with a child for the sexual gratification of an adult or caretaker. This includes exposure of child to sexual acts or materials, inappropriate touch, or any other sexual contact between the child and caretaker.*

PHYSICAL INDICATORS OF SEXUAL ABUSE OF THE VICTIM

* Pain or itching of the anal or genital areas
* Blood stained underwear
* Bedwetting
* Sexually transmitted diseases
* Penile or vaginal discharge
* Pregnancy
* Difficulty with walking or sitting
* Injuries or bruises of the genital areas
* Obesity

BEHAVIORAL INDICATORS OF SEXUAL ABUSE OF THE VICTIM

* Promiscuity
* Withdrawal
* Extreme modesty
* Runs away from home and/or from people
* Poor peer-relationships
* Seductiveness
* Bizarre or sophisticated behavior
* Self destructive behavior
* Low self-esteem
* Eating disturbances
* Sleep disturbances
* Nightmares
* Guilt and shame

BEHAVIORAL INDICATORS OF CARETAKERS

* Alcohol and drug problems
* Feelings of inadequacy
* Breakdown of adult intimate relationships
* Role confusion
* History of victimization
* Inadequate social skills
* Domestic violence
* Problems with impulse control

Protect Against Child Abuse

THINK ABUSE

1. *Sexually transmitted diseases*

2. *Difficulty walking*

3. *Eating disturbances*

4. *Seductive*

5. *The caretaker may have a history of victimization*

6. *Domestic violence*

NEGLECT

Neglect is defined as *the failure of the caretaker to provide adequate food, clothing, shelter, medical attention and protection to such a degree that the child's well being or development is likely to be significantly damaged.*

PHYSICAL INDICATORS OF THE VICTIM

* Constant hunger
* Weight loss
* Inappropriate dress or clothing
* Lack of supervision
* Poor hygiene
* Constant fatigue
* Chronic illness without medical attention
* Developmental delays

BEHAVIORAL INDICATORS OF THE VICTIM

* Begging
* Stealing food
* Sleeping in school
* Delinquency
* Runaway
* Truancy
* Alcohol and or drug abuse
* Extreme behaviors

BEHAVIORAL INDICATORS OF THE CAREGIVER

* Emotional problems
* Financial problems
* Drug and alcohol problems
* Limited parenting skills
* History of mental illness
* Intellectual limitations
* Refusal to comply with medical recommendations
* Failure to attend school conferences

Protect Against Child Abuse

THINK ABUSE

1. Inappropriate dress

2. Poor hygiene

3. Sleeping in school

4. Stealing food

5. Parents may have limited parenting skills

CHAPTER FOUR

PHYSICAL ASSESSMENT OF THE "NORMAL" CHILD

This section of the book will describe the assessment of the *"normal"* child. In the context of this text, *"normal"* will be defined *as no clearly identifiable abnormalities or deformities.* If, at any time during the assessment, there is any question about *"normal"* vs. *"abnormal"* findings, a medical evaluation should be considered.

ASSESSMENT OF THE CHILD "HEAD TO TOE"

HEAD

round
symmetrical
child is alert and awake

NOSE

normal in shape and size

EYES

clear
no drainage
no redness

EARS

normal placement
no drainage
no pain

LIPS

intact
without injury

HAIR

normal texture
normal distribution

CHEST

equal rise and fall
regular rate and rhythm
no difficulty breathing
no deformities of the chest or ribs noted

ABDOMEN

flat
soft
no pain
no changes in voiding
no pain when voiding
no changes in stool

EXTREMITIES

able to move without pain
able to stand and bear weight
straight alignment
appears developmentally appropriate

SKIN

    warm
    dry
    no rashes
    no discoloration
    no swelling

GENITALIA

    normal female or male
    no discharge
    no bleeding
    no pain
    no swelling
    no discoloration

Normal Placement of Internal Organs for a School Age Child

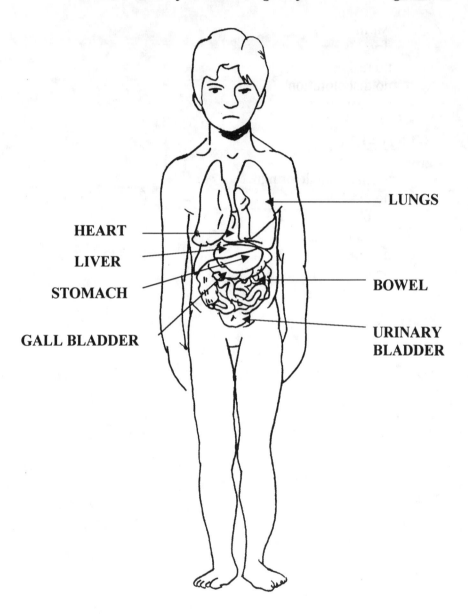

HEART

LIVER

STOMACH

GALL BLADDER

LUNGS

BOWEL

URINARY
BLADDER

Normal Skeletal System – Frontal View

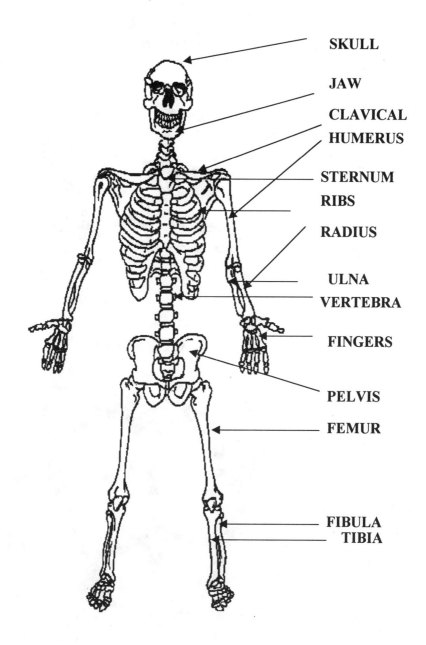

SKULL

JAW

CLAVICAL

HUMERUS

STERNUM

RIBS

RADIUS

ULNA

VERTEBRA

FINGERS

PELVIS

FEMUR

FIBULA

TIBIA

Top and Side Views of the Skull

ANTERIOR FONTENELL
(SOFT SPOT)

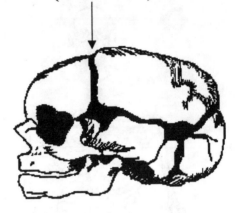

BACK OF SKULL

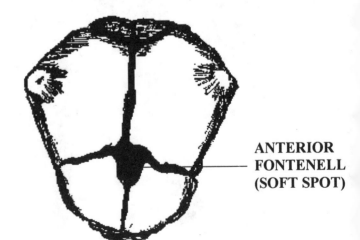

ANTERIOR FONTENELL (SOFT SPOT)

FRONT OF SKULL

CHAPTER FIVE

CHILD ABUSE INJURIES

FRACTURES

A fracture may be defined as a *complete or incomplete break in the bone or cartilage*. Some types of fractures are more frequently associated with abuse because of the mechanism of injury. Fractures are often found only when the child is brought to the hospital for other reasons. Long bone fractures are the most commonly inflicted fractures and skull fractures are the second most common.

Fractures can result from a number of mechanisms of injury including pushing, shoving, pulling, twisting, punching, grabbing, hitting or shaking.

Although many of the fractures described here can happen throughout childhood, this discussion will address these fractures as they relate to abuse.

- ## SPIRAL FRACTURE and OBLIQUE FRACTURE

DESCRIPTION: A spiral fracture is a twisted fracture.

MECHANISM OF INJURY: Spiral and oblique fractures have similar mechanisms of injury. They can be caused by violently jerking or twisting of a limb. Children that are non-ambulatory are very unlikely to sustain this type of fracture as a result of an accident. It is common that the caregiver will say that the child twisted his or her leg in the crib side rail which is not the mechanism nor force required to cause this injury.

Examples of a Spiral Fracture and Oblique Fracture

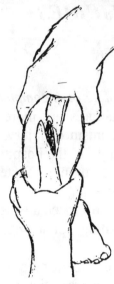

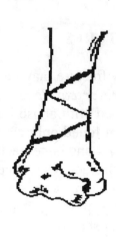

Spiral Fracture
(Twisting of the extremity)

Spiral Fracture

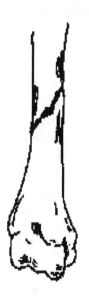

Oblique Fracture

- **SIMPLE OR CLOSED FRACTURE**

    DESCRIPTION: A simple or closed fracture is a fracture of the bone where there is no injury to the skin at the sight of the fracture.

    MECHANISM OF INJURY: This is a very common childhood fracture. It can be caused by falls or blunt force. Although it is a common fracture, abuse should be considered when the history is inconsistent with the injury.

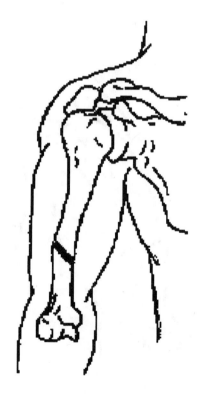

Simple or Closed Fracture

- **COMPOUND OR OPEN FRACTURE**

  DESCRIPTION: A compound or open fracture is one which has injury to the skin at the site of the fracture. In some cases with this type of fracture there may be a piece of bone protruding through the skin.

  MECHANISM OF INJURY: A compound fracture is often related to abuse when there is a significant and violent blunt force.

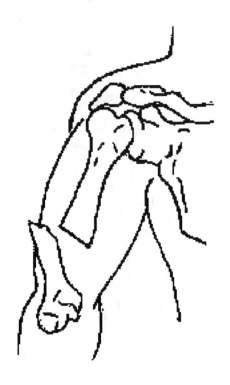

Compound or Open Fracture

- ## COMMINUTED FRACTURE

  DESCRIPTION: A comminuted fracture is described when the bone shatters and there is skin and tissue injury at the site of the fracture.

  MECHANISM OF INJURY: A comminuted fracture would require severe violent force to the bone area. In the absence of a motor vehicle accident or similar event this type of fracture is highly suspicious of abuse.

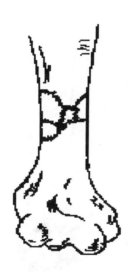

Comminuted Fracture

- **TRANSVERSE FRACTURE**

    DESCRIPTION: Transverse fracture is a fracture that crosses the entire shaft of the bone.

    MECHANISM OF INJURY: A blunt force is required to produce this type of fracture. Abuse is suspected when the history is not consistent with the injury. A common history offered would be that the child ran into a table. A child is not able to generate the force by him or herself to inflict this type of injury.

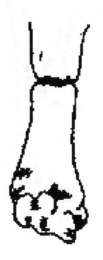

Transverse Fracture

- **EPIPHYSEAL-METAPHYSEAL FRACTURE**

  DESCRIPTION: This type of fracture is usually caused by pulling or twisting of the limb resulting in a fracture located at the growth plate.

  MECHANISM OF INJURY: A sudden violent pulling and/or twisting of the limb is necessary to cause this type of fracture. These types of fractures are generally indicative of abuse in children preschool or younger.

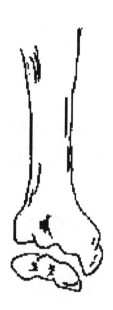

Epiphyseal-Metaphyseal Fracture

- **IMPACTED FRACTURE**

    DESCRIPTION: A fracture that occurs when a fragment of the bone is forcefully driven into another bone.

    MECHANSIM OF INJURY: This type of fracture is related to severe violence. Child abuse should be suspected when there is no significant or plausible history available. This injury can occur when a child is violently made to sit with repeated and forceful impact causing impact fractures of the spine.

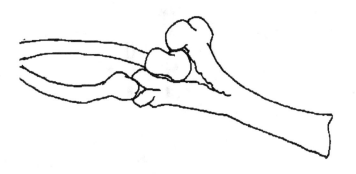

Impacted Fracture

• <u>RIB FRACTURES</u>

DESCRIPTION: The ribs are located in the chest and back providing a protective cage for the organs that lie beneath. Fractures of the rib cage can be simple or compound just as any other bone. Due to the resilience the rib cage it is very difficult to fracture a rib in children.

MECHANISM OF INJURY: Rib fractures are usually caused by a significant direct blow or crushing force. When rib fractures are found in children under one year, Shaken Baby Syndrome should be considered.

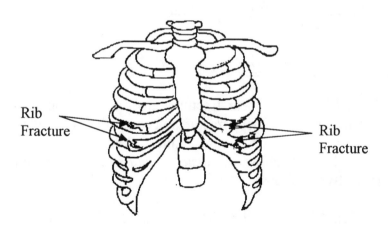

Rib
Fracture

Rib
Fracture

<u>Multiple Fractures of the Ribs</u>

- ## SKULL FRACTURE

  DESCRIPTION: The skull is defined as the bony structure of the head. The bones of the skull are not completely fused at the time of the birth. This makes it possible for the head to pass through the birth canal. There are two fontanels – "soft spots" – at the time of birth and by eighteen months both "soft spots" have closed. The most rapid growth in the skull occurs during the first seven years of life.

  MECHANISM OF INJURY: There are two types of skull fractures of which the linear skull fracture is the most common. The *linear skull fracture* occurs at the point of injury and may spread from that point to different directions.

  The second type of fracture is known as a *depressed skull fracture*. The skull bone is forced inward and may cause injury to the underlying tissues and brain.

- ## LINEAR FRACTURES

  DESCRIPTION: Linear fractures are fractures that present in a line formation. Linear fractures occur at the point of injury and can often spread or radiate. Linear skull fractures that cross a suture line are known as *diastatic skull fractures* which are more indicative of abuse.

  MECHANISM OF INJURY: Linear skull fractures are very common in childhood. These fractures can be accidental, caused by motor vehicle accidents or falls. If the history is not consistent, you should then suspect abuse. In most cases of abuse there will be other signs of abuse in conjunction with the fracture. With infants you must review and carefully evaluate the child for a history of abuse. Any type of blunt trauma to the head may cause linear fractures in abuse.

- **DEPRESSED SKULL FRACTURES**

    DESCRIPTION: Depressed skull fractures occur when severe blunt force is applied to the skull causing a depression in the bone, which may intrude into the brain. This type of fracture is the more severe of the two. The fracture, depending on its location, can cause damage and bleeding into the brain.

    MECHANISM OF INJURY: Depressed skull fractures are caused when the head is hit or forced into an object. An example would be the head being hit with a bat, phone, bottle or other hard object. A child being thrown or pushed forcefully into a protruding solid object may also cause a depressed skull fracture.

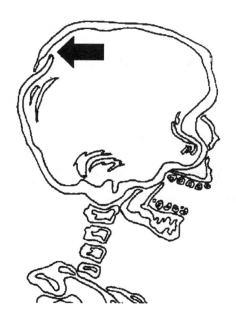

Side View of the Skull
(Arrow Indicated a Depressed Skull Fracture)

Protect Against Child Abuse

THINK ABUSE

1. *Spiral fractures in non-ambulatory children*

2. *Fractures in various stages of healing*

3. *Rib fractures in children under one year of age*

4. *Diastatic and/or depressed skull fractures*

5. *Inconsistent history related to the injury*

CHAPTER SIX

HEAD INJURIES

Head injuries are the most common cause of death or permanent disability resulting from child abuse. The majority of head injuries during the first year of life are the result of physical abuse. Children under the age of two are at high risk for injuries secondary to blows or violent shaking. In most cases, there is a significant discrepancy between the history and the physical findings when evaluating for child abuse.

SHAKEN BABY SYNDROME (SBS)

Shaken Baby Syndrome (also known as Whiplash Shaken Infant Syndrome) is most frequently seen in children under the age of one. Children under one year are at risk due to the lack of strength of the neck muscles and the disproportionately large head. Shaken Baby Syndrome results when a child is shaken, causing the brain to be forced forward and backward against the unmoving skull. This force causes the bridging arteries and veins within the brain to rupture causing bleeding in the brain and skull. In most cases these infants present to the hospital in an unconscious state with no history of injury. They may also present with seizures, abnormally low body temperature and abnormal respirations. The caretaker's history often indicates that no medical professional had been consulted regarding early signs of injury. These early signs may include vomiting, lethargy, irritably and a decrease in muscle tone or floppiness. There may also be retinal hemorrhage or bleeding in the eyes. There may be no other signs of injury.

DESCRIPTION: When evaluating Shaken Baby Syndrome there are four points to remember:

1. A child may have been shaken some time prior to presentation in the emergency room. The child may be critically ill or unconscious at the time of presentation.

2. Due to the child's age, the fontanels are not closed and the sutures lines are not fused thus allowing for brain swelling with only early signs of brain injury.

3. The caretaker may have previously brought the child to a medical professional for vomiting and/or irritability with no history of significant head trauma, indicating the possibility of original time of injury.

4. Occasionally there will be signs of other abuse associated with shaken baby such as finger print bruises (known as grab marks) where they were held and/or facial bruising. Although there are these occasional cases where bruising or other injuries are present it remains prudent to obtain a complete skeletal survey to evaluate for additional fractures or injuries.

MECHANISM OF INJURY: Violent shaking of infant allowing the head to bob.

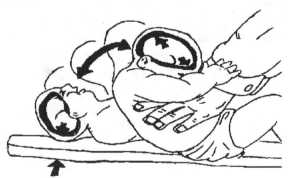

Shaken Baby Syndrome

HEMORRAGES AND HEMATOMAS

Hemorrhage is the term used to describe *active bleeding*. *Hematoma* is the term used to describe *the pooling or collection of blood in a space or cavity.*

Intercranial pressure is defined as *the normal pressure in the brain produced by the cerebrospinal fluid.*

When blood pools or collects in the brain it increases the intercranial pressure. The signs of increased intercranial pressure are headache, vomiting, irritability, lethargy, changes in consciousness, (i.e. increased sleeping), seizures, bulging fontanel, personality or behavioral changes, dizziness, and death.

• SUBDURAL HEMORRHAGE

DESCRIPTION: Subdural hemorrhage or hematoma occurs when there is bleeding into the subdural space in the brain. Subdural hemorrhage is caused by the breaking or severing of the large veins. This breaking of the veins occurs with the motion of the brain hitting the skull. The subdural space does not have the capacity to absorb blood readily thus causing increased intercranial pressure.

MECHANISM OF INJURY: A blow to the front or back of the head that causes a rapid acceleration of the brain against the skull. In shaken baby syndrome, the rapid acceleration or deceleration of the brain against the skull may cause a subdural hemorrhage.

Also known to occur in birth trauma, noting that symptoms usually will occur within 24-48 hours.

- ## EPIDURAL HEMORRHAGE

  DESCRIPTION: Epidural Hemorrhages are caused by a blow to the side of the skull causing bleeding between the dura matter and the membrane covering the skull (the periosteum). This injury may cause a loss of consciousness but the child may recover after the initial phase. This also causes changes in intercranial pressure.

  MECHANISMS OF INJURY: Blows or blunt trauma to the side of the head.

- ## SUBGALEAL HEMORRHAGE

  DESCRIPTION: Bleeding between the scalp and the skull.

  MECHANISMS OF INJURY: Traumatic alopecia is when there is violent hair pulling resulting in areas of baldness. Violent hair pulling with or without loss of hair can also cause subgaleal hemorrhage. In both cases bruising or swelling in the area of the scalp can be noted.

- ## RETINAL HEMORRHAGE

  DESCRIPTION: This is a term used to describe bleeding in the back of the eye known as the retina. Retinal hemorrhaging takes ten to fourteen days to clear. Evaluation and diagnosis of this injury is made by a fundoscopic exam. The causes of retinal hemorrhage can be from the sudden compression of the chest, shaking, head trauma, high blood pressure and bleeding disorders.

  MECHANISMS OF INJURY: Shaken Baby Syndrome (SBS) is frequently associated with retinal hemorrhages.

Sudden compression of the chest, usually a result of motor vehicle impact, versus the result of chest compressions during CPR.

Twirling on the horizontal bar as a gymnastics

Rarely seen in accidental head injury, child abuse should be considered

Protect Against Child Abuse

THINK ABUSE

1. Shaken Baby Syndrome

2. Bleeding in the brain not associated with significant history

3. Retinal hemorrhages

CHAPTER SEVEN

SKIN INJURIES

This section will discuss skin injuries and the common terms used to describe and define these injuries. *A skin injury is the change or changes in the appearance of the skin.* There are many forms of skin injuries that occur and many words that can be used to describe them.

Abrasion is a scrape, or skinned knee or injury such as a rug burn. There is minimal bleeding in this type of injury.

Laceration is the ripping of the skin, also known as a "cut". This can also be a puncture or penetrating wound such as a stab. Bleeding will depend on the severity and depth of the wound.

Bruise is the black and blue mark seen on the skin. Bruises can also be called *ecchymosis* or *contusion.* Bruises are usually caused by a blunt force causing the superficial blood vessels under the skin to break causing discoloration. The surface of the skin remains intact, and there is no external bleeding.

Edema is the collection of fluid or swelling in the tissues or skin. Edema can be caused by bumps, bruises, allergic reactions, illness, or other injury.

Skin injuries are the most common form of injury in child abuse. Skin injuries such as bruises, cuts and scrapes are the most easily identified. Young children especially children in their toddler years will have bruises over the bony prominences such as the shin, knee, elbow and forehead. On the other hand these are the same children that are at highest risk for child abuse. It is important to familiarize yourself with an understanding of child development in order to understand and evaluate the caretakers history regarding bruises or other injuries. It is important for you to understand at what age a child is able to master certain activities such as rolling, walking or climbing. For example, a child of one month of age "rolling off the dressing table", is clearly not within developmental age appropriateness. Children, during the toddler years, frequently fall when learning to walk, and you would expect to see bruises on the knees and shins. It would not be appropriate for a child of this age to have bruises on the buttocks, abdomen or cheeks.

Although skin injuries are common indicators of abuse there are a number of medical explanations and or illnesses that can cause skin injuries. Some of these illnesses include, but are not limited to:

- Hemophilia
- Idiopathic thrombocytopenia
- Anemia
- Leukemia

A medical evaluation will assist in differentiating these illnesses from abuse.

Other explanations of discoloration of the skin can be related to birth marks, such as stork bites, Mongolian spots and strawberry marks.

LOCATION

Some of the more common locations of skin injuries that would lead you to suspect abuse are as follows:

MOUTH INJURIES

The mouth is frequently a location for inflicted injuries usually due to inappropriate feeding, a childs inability to communicate and/or crying. Bottles, eating utensils, gags, hands or fingers and/or blunt trauma, inflict most inflicted trauma. Skin injuries that may result are cuts, scrapes, bruises, chafing and/or loss of teeth. A frequent injury of the mouth is a tear of the frenulum. The frenulum is the piece of skin that connects the lips to the gums and the tongue to the floor of the mouth. Injury to the frenulum is most frequently caused by forcing a bottle, pacifier of spoon into the child's mouth.

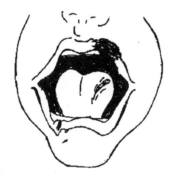

**Injuries to the mouth may include laceration of the tongue
and laceration and bruising of the lips**

EAR INJURIES

Pulling, pinching or a direct blow usually causes injury to the ear. Bruising behind the ear known as *"battle sign"* can be indicative of a more serious head injury. If a child suffers a direct blow to the ear it may cause the ear drum to rupture.

EYE INJURIES

Conjunctival hemorrhage is the pooling of blood in the white portion of the eyes caused by inflicted injury or blunt force.

Acute hyphema is the pooling of the blood in the colored section of the eyes. The causes are by inflicted injury or blunt force.

Black eyes also known as *periorbital ecchymosis* is swelling and bruising around the eye. This is the most common type of inflicted injury. Black eyes in children are not common accidental injuries and the presence of two black eyes should increase your suspicion of abuse.

Retinal hemorrhage is bleeding behind the retina. This type of eye injury is often seen as a result of inflicted head injuries such as Shaken Baby Syndrome.

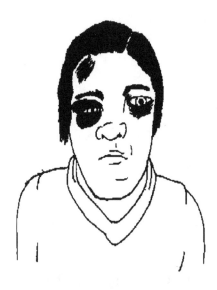

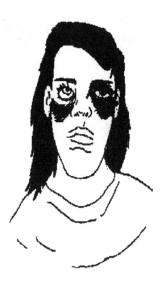

Swelling-discoloration, especially around the eyes and additional head injury is suspect when no history or an inappropriate history is given.

Orbit fractures should be suspected when there is limited upward gaze. Abuse Should be suspected without appropriate history or medical condition.

BACK, CHEST and ABDOMINAL INJURIES

Back, chest and abdominal bruising is rarely accidental due to the force of impact needed to cause bruising. If the history is of an accidental nature it must include a fall onto a blunt object. Injuries in this area could be related to hitting (with or without objects), punching or squeezing. If injuries to this area are observed, internal injuries may also be present. Further medical evaluation is needed.

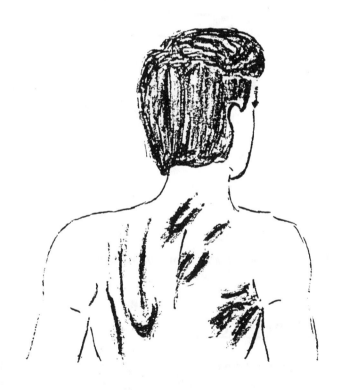

Bruising to back with noted patterns are very suspect of abuse.

BUTTOCKS and THIGH

Buttocks and thigh injuries are frequent sights of inflicted injury. Due to the fleshy and muscular make up of these areas the force required to cause bruising would be significant or extreme. The inflicted injury is usually caused by the child being kicked or hit with an object such as a strap, cord or stick.

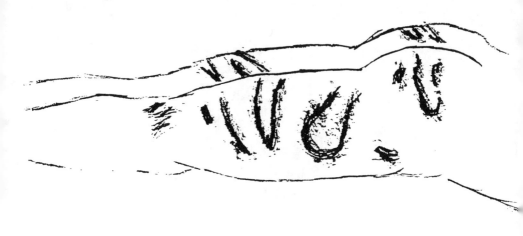

Bruising, both old and new noted, same pattern marks also noted are very suspect of abuse

NORMAL BRUISING

Shins, knees and arms are common sites of injuries that are related to accidents or normal childhood injuries. Although these sites are common areas of bruising for children, bizarre marks and excessive bruising indicates the need to investigate further.

TYPES OF SKIN INJIRIES

The types of injuries in an abusive situation can lead to identifiable marks. The list of information that follows includes, but is not limited to, a number of marks or injuries that are commonly seen in abusive situations.

BRUISES

When numerous bruises of various ages are seen this could be indicative of abuse. The age and color of the bruises are dependent on a number of factors including skin color, rate of healing, the extent of broken vessels under the skin and the distance of the injury from the surface of the skin. The color change in the healing process is as follows:

Initially a bruise will be reddish-blue-purple changing to a greenish-yellow then fading further to brown until it completely fades away.

Some other commonly seen bruises can be from pinching and grabbing. Grab marks are usually oval in shape resembling finger tips. They are commonly seen on the upper torso, arms and cheeks from forcefully restraining or shaking a child.

PATTERN and BIZARRE MARKS

Pattern marks are usually pathomonic of abuse. Frequently disciplinary measures have left pattern marks. These marks are identified by the object used to inflict abuse. It is necessary to measure the width and length of these marks to assist in identifying the object used. Some specific pattern or bizarre marks include, but are not limited to:

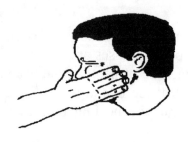 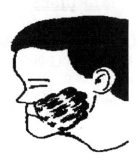

Slap marks to face bruising and redness caused by facial skin and tissue squeezed between hand and finger

LOOP MARKS

Loop marks are usually caused by a cord or rope that has been doubled over to be used to hit the child. Cords or ropes used in this way are commonly utilized for disciplinary reasons. These marks can cause bruises, swelling, lacerations and abrasions. Based on the location of these injuries, medical evaluation may need to be completed to rule out underlying internal injuries.

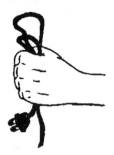 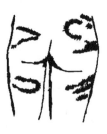

Loop marks made with an extension cord

PATTERN MARK ILLUSTRATION

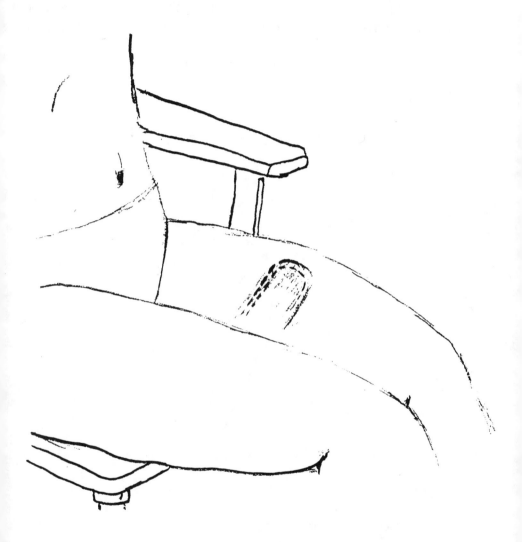

Belt mark on the inner thigh noting a clear pattern of the belt stitiching

PADDLE MARKS

Paddle marks are another patter mark that can be observed on a child. These marks can range from spoon, shoe or brush shape, each producing its own specific pattern. An example of this would be a brush leaving a rectangular shape with bristal marks.

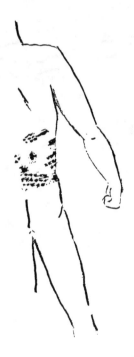

Wire Brush Pattern

LINEAR MARKS

Linear marks are characterized by a horizontal or vertical lines. They can cause welts, bruises, lacerations and abrasions. A number of objects can cause linear marks such as a ruler, model train track, stick or "switch".

LIGATURE MARKS

Ligature marks are encircling tie marks usually found on the wrist, arm, leg, ankle, waist or neck, indicating the child has been forcibly restrained. These injuries are generally caused by using fishing string, rope or cord and may cause a deep laceration to the area tied.

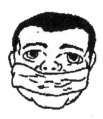 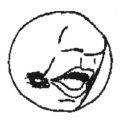

Bruises, swelling and redness as seen in the binding of a child's mouth.

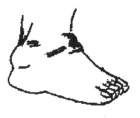

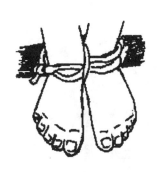

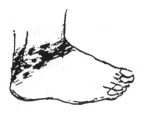

Child bound at the ankles with resulting swelling and blistering

BITE MARKS

Human bite marks are found in both physical and sexual abuse. When evaluating human bite marks, measurements can be taken to identify the perpetrator. Measurement greater than three centimeters indicates an adult bite where as less then three centimeters indicate a child's bite. The evaluation of bite marks is best made by a forensic dentist and if abuse is suspected, a forensic dentist should be consulted.

Location of bite marks are frequently found on the back and arms.

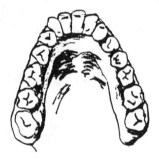

Approximate normal size – greater than 3cm from canine to canine

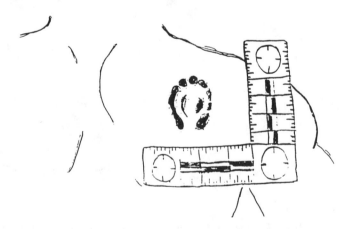

Bite marks on a childs back drawn with a right angle ruler
Use of a ruler is very important for purposes of sizing the wound

Protect Against Child Abuse

THINK ABUSE

1. *Location of marks*

2. *Definable pattern*

3. *Bruises and swelling*

4. *Developmentally inappropriate injury*

5. *Multiple stages of healing*

6. *Statement from child*

CHAPTER EIGHT

BURNS

Burns can happen in any household. The location and severity of the burn and the amount of time that passes before medical attention is sought will assist in delineating between accidental and non accidental burns. Most burns are preventable accidents, however, they may also be inflicted injuries used as punishment. Children under the age of five are most often the victims of burns. When a child is brought to the attention of the medical professionals, other abusive injuries are often present. The most frequent accidental burns are from hot liquids spilling on the child. Most of these burns are located on the head, neck, chest, stomach and arms.

Burn abuse frequently centers around toileting, bedwetting and soiling. The most common sites of abusive burns are the hands, legs, feet, buttock and genital areas. Burns are described as first, second cr third degree and measured by the percentage of the body burned.

First degree burns are similar to a sun burn. The external layer of the skin is reddened, swollen and tender. This type of burn will peel but no scarring occurs.

Second degree burns damage the first and second layers of the skin, expose the nerve endings and cause them to be very painful. Blistering is common but these burns normally heal without scars.

Third degree burns damage the skin and the tissue beneath. These are also called full thickness burns. The appearance of a third degree burn is white or charred accompanied by massive blistering. With full thickness burns sensation is lost in these areas. Full thickness or third degree burns leave scarring, disrupt normal body functioning and frequently require skin grafts as treatment.

All burns regardless of degree can be life threatening depending on the percentage of the body burned. There are a number of different types of abusive burns in children. The urgent nature of the injury sometimes takes precedence over obtaining a good history. The burns discussed are the most common types of burns in child abuse.

Normal Skin Layers

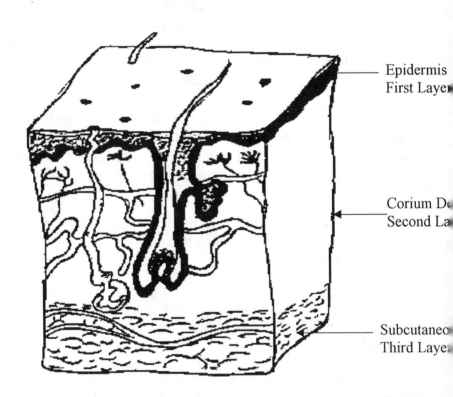

Epidermis
First Layer

Corium De
Second La

Subcutaneo
Third Layer

CONTACT BURNS

Contact burns occur when the skin is placed in contact with hot metal objects such as heater grates, curling irons, clothes irons and stoves or stove burners. Most of these burns form an image of the object. For example, a child's back placed on a hot heater grate would show linear burn marks that resemble the pattern of the heater grate. Other contact burns can occur from cigarettes, cigars or caustic substances. One of the most common types of contact burns is a cigarette burn that presents in a circular pattern measuring seven to eight millimeters. The most common location for a cigarette burn is generally on the hands, arms or feet. Cigarette burns are usually multiple and similar in size and depth.

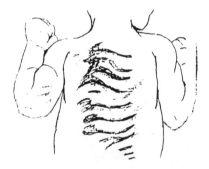

Contact burn to the back caused by a child being held on a heating grate

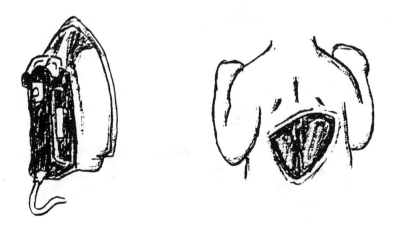

Burn to the back caused by a clothing iron being held on the child's back

CONTACT BURNS

<u>Cigarette Burn Patterns</u>

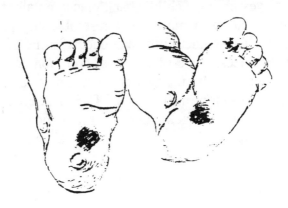

Cigarette burn to the bottom of the feet in varying degrees of burn injury

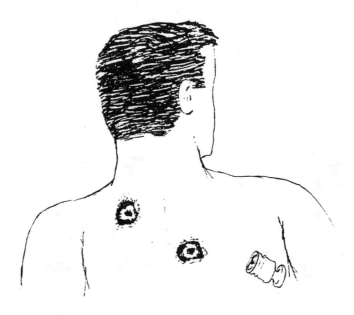

Burn patterns to the back caused by a cigarette lighter from a car

<u>Cigarette Burn Patterns</u>

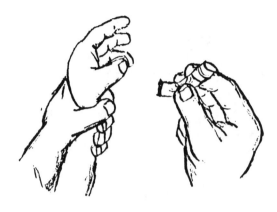

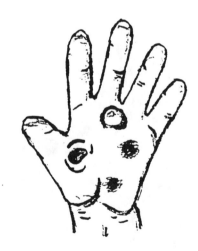

Cigarette burns to the palm of the hand

SCALDING BURNS

Burns that are a result of scalding are the most frequent cause of thermal injury in child abuse. Scalds are caused by hot liquid on the skin. Scald burns from tap water are more severe and extensive than from an injury such as spilling coffee on the child. Most often these injuries occur when the caretaker is in the same room as the child, although the history from the caretaker may indicate they left the child alone for a short period of time.

The extent of the burns from hot tap water depend on the water temperature and exposure time. Most homes and apartment buildings have water temperatures set at 130 degrees or greater. Exposure to water temperature of 130 degrees requires only thirty seconds to cause a full thickness burn. Temperature of 158 degrees requires only one second to cause a scald burn.

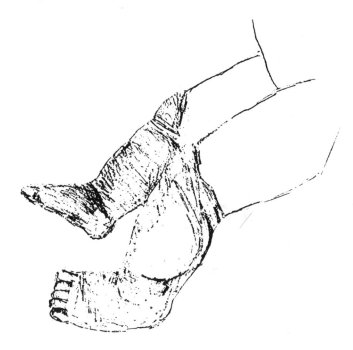

Burns of the lower legs - *"stocking"* burn pattern

IMMERSION BURNS

Immersion burns are a type of scald burn that results from a child being forcefully immersed in hot liquid such as water in a bath tub. Immersion burns cause a uniform burn line called the line of demarcation. Which is the line marking the separation between the area burned and the area that has not been burned. The area of the skin that is spared is usually the buttocks which has been pressed against the bottom of the tub, causing a donut shaped area or pattern. Other characteristic patterns of immersion burns is flexion. When a child is immersed into hot water he will flex or pull his knees to his chest in an attempt to guard himself. The area of skin spared is between the folds and creases of the thighs, genital area and possibly a small section of the lower abdomen.

Other types of immersion burns are caused when a child's hands or feet are dunked into hot liquid. These types of burns have very characteristic patterns called stocking burns of the feet, and gloved burns of the hands. This is very suggestible of abuse because usually both legs or hands are burned identically.

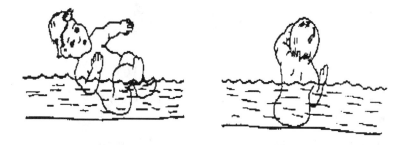

Descriptive drawing showing how the child is dunked in hot water and demonstrating the areas that would be burned

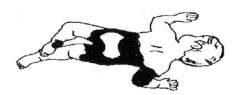

Area of the skin that is spared - buttocks shows donut pattern of sparing

FILICIDE

Filicide refers to cases in which a child is murdered by fire and the caretaker is the perpetrator. Although this is considered rare, it is the ultimate form of child abuse. Filicide occurs when a child is locked or forcibly restrained and the dwelling is set on fire.

Protect Against Child Abuse

THINK ABUSE

1. *Children under five years are most often victims*

2. *Location of abusive burns are on hands, legs, feet, buttocks, and genital areas*

3. *Contact burns especially with a definable pattern*

4. *Inconsistent history*

5. *Lines of demarcation, sparing, donut shaped burns*

CHAPTER NINE

CHEST AND ABDOMINAL INJURIES

Injuries to the chest can be caused by blunt or squeezing trauma and can often be associated with fractures of the ribs, causing perforated or bruised lungs. These types of injuries may present themselves as pain in the chest wall or back, difficulty ambulating and difficulty breathing.

Abdominal injuries are the second most common cause of death in inflicted injuries. Children under the age of three are at the most risk of death. Some of the common factors that cause death of a child from an abdominal injury include the fact that the distance between the stomach and spine is much shorter, the liver is larger relative to the size of the child, and the muscles surrounding and protecting the abdominal cavity are thinner and much less rigid than that of an adult. In children the rib cage protects less of the abdominal cavity than that of an adult. The internal organs found in the abdominal cavity are the spleen, liver, pancreas, stomach, kidneys, and intestines. Injuries to the abdominal area can cause ruptures, tears, perforations or bruising (hematomas.) The type of injury inflicted will depend on where the injury occurred and by what means. When there is blunt trauma applied to the abdomen and depending on the placement of the injury, the organ injured can be identified.

Blunt trauma may be defined as *a kick or punch with significant force.* The type of injuries listed below are commonly found in blunt trauma. As always the professional must evaluate the history of the injury to assess if it fits the type of injury involved. In most cases of accidental injury to the abdominal cavity, other injuries to the long bones, head and chest will be present.

A rupture or perforation of the stomach or the intestines may be seen if the blunt trauma occurs over this area. To clarify, these are hollow organs, and can be compared to a balloon that is secured, being punched or kicked forcefully, causing it to pop.

Trauma to the solid organs such as the liver and pancreas can cause injuries such as tears and lacerations. Forceful blunt trauma to these organs can cause the organ to tear or rip causing internal and rapid bleeding.

All organs can be bruised causing hematomas. The most common site of hematomas is the jejunum, and duodenum (part of the intestine). The child may also suffer bruising to any of the other organs from forceful trauma.

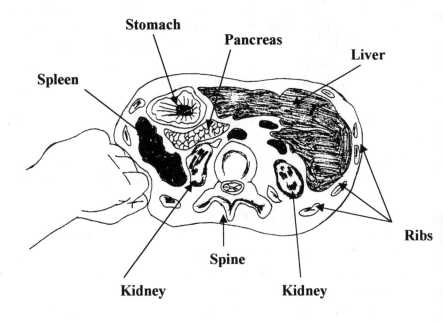

Normal anatomy of the abdomen
Punch - indicating the possible injury that can be caused by forceful blows

Illustrations Blunt Injuries

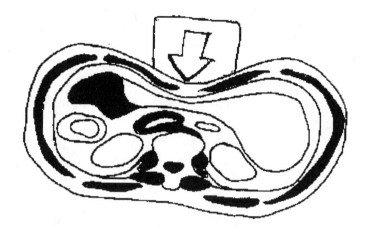

Blunt injury demonstrating potential crushing of internal organs against the vertebrae

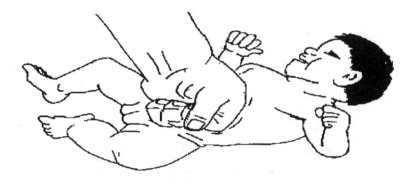

Blunt injury to infant from an adult fist

Injuries to the abdominal cavity can also be caused when forceful trauma is applied to the back. An example of this would be a blunt trauma to the kidney area that would cause a kidney fracture. A kidney fracture is equivalent to a tear or laceration of the kidney.

External examination may or may not reveal bruising. The child's abdomen is frequently swollen and tender. Nausea and vomiting may also be present. These types of injuries can be lethal and death can occur rapidly.

Protect Against Child Abuse

THINK ABUSE

1. *Children under the age of three are at greatest risk of death*

2. *Chest pain, difficulty ambulating, difficulty breathing*

3. *Not necessarily able to see bruising*

4. *History not consistent*

5. *The abuser must be larger than the victim.*

CHAPTER TEN

GENITAL INJURIES

Injuries to the genital area can occur due to physical and/ or sexual abuse. Injuries related to physical abuse can range from superficial skin trauma to internal injuries.

Physical abuse injuries are usually related to toilet training or "accidents" when a child "wets his/her pants". Some of the common injuries seen due to toilet training in boys are a bruised penis, testicular ruptures, scrotal tears and ligature marks around the penis. In females it is more common to see vaginal bruising from pinching of the labia, kicking and or hitting the area, swelling of the area related to any of the above stated injuries and infection. Other physical injuries to the genitalia may be related to a caretakers rage with a child. Although it may be difficult to differentiate between sexual assault and physical abuse, it is necessary to obtain a detailed history of the events leading up to the injury.

A child may present with internal injuries due to some type of object being inserted into the vagina or anus. This type of injury may have no relation to sexual assault but be an attempt by an enraged caretaker to prevent the child from further soiling in a diaper or bed. It may also be a punishment of the child due to masturbation or "playing with themselves". This type of injury is not meant for the sexual gratification of the adult but as punishment to the child for a behavior that is not acceptable to the adult.

Injuries to the genitalia related to sexual assault can be very similar to those of physical abuse. These injuries in females may include, but not limited to, vaginal tearing, abrasions, lacerations and bruises of the outer aspect of the vagina (labia majora). The inner aspect of the vaginal area (labia minora), may show changes in vascularity, scarring, and changes in shape and size. In males there may be injuries related to bite marks, bruising of the scrotal area, swelling of the tip of the penis, or swelling of the urethra (opening where urine is expelled).

There are a number of signs and symptoms that are associated with injuries to the genitalia. Some of these symptoms are discharge from the penis or vaginal area, swelling, pain, itching, foul odor, difficulty urinating, or pain upon urination and bleeding. Some of the indicators the child may present with are pain when sitting, difficulty sitting, difficulty walking, incontinence of urine and/or stool, and behavioral changes. Upon medical evaluation the child may be found to have sexually transmitted diseases such as HIV, gonorrhea, syphilis, chlamydia, herpes and venereal warts. The child may also be pregnant.

Not all sexually transmitted diseases are indicative of abuse. Some of these diseases may be passed to the child during the birth process. This is a situation that must be evaluated by a medical professional trained in child sexual assault.

Injuries to the anus can occur in both the male and female child. These injures will appear the same in both sexes. Injuries that are evidence of abuse may include tears, scars, abrasions, swelling, and bruising. When chronic abuse is present the sphincter tone is lost. Loss of sphincter tone may result in staining of the underwear by stool. Staining alone is not diagnostic of chronic abuse. A detailed history and interview of the child and corroborating information should be present to make a complete evaluation.

Illustrations of Genital Injuries

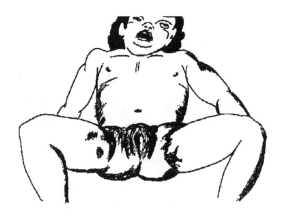

Female child presenting with extensive swelling, bruising and injury to the gentalia and inner thighs

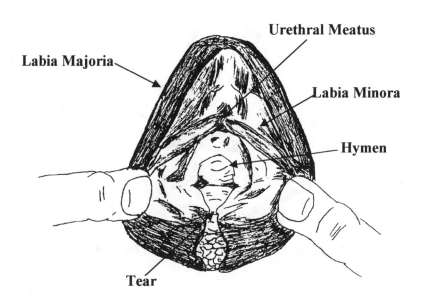

Laceration of internal female anatomy

<u>Illustrations Gential Injuries</u>

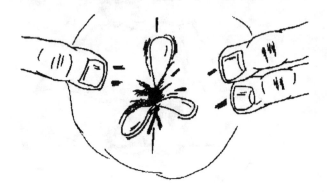

Male child presenting with acute anal injury

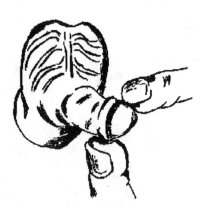

Pinching of the penis causing brusing and swelling

Protect Against Child Abuse

THINK ABUSE

1. *Can be physical or sexual abuse*

2. *Unrealistic toilet training expectations*

3. *Burning upon urination*

4. *Pain when sitting*

5. *Bleeding*

6. *Change in behavior*

CHAPTER ELEVEN

FAILURE TO THRIVE

Failure to thrive is defined as *the abnormally slow growth and development of a child.* Most children who suffer from failure to thrive are under the age of two years.

There are three distinct forms of failure to thrive:

1. **<u>Organic failure to thrive</u>** is related to a disease process that causes a child to experience poor weight gain

2. **<u>Inorganic failure to thrive</u>** is related to a lack of parenting skills, maternal deprivation, or the lack of adequate nutrition

3. **<u>Mixed failure to thrive</u>** is related to an underlying disease process that requires an increased caloric intake that the caretaker is unable to provide. The caretaker may be unaware of the child's increased needs.

The diagnosis of failure to thrive is made by a medical professional based on standardized growth curves. These growth curves indicate the expected growth in height, weight and head circumference at specific ages of the child. In the diagnosis of failure to thrive a child will be below the fifth percentile in height, weight or head circumference. Each child has their own specific growth curve. An indication of failure to thrive would be a significant loss in any one of the three stated areas.

In diagnosing failure to thrive there are a number of areas that need to be evaluated both medically and socially. These areas are listed below.

Areas of Assessment in Failure to Thrive

- Medical evaluation to rule out underlying disease
- History of acute illness
- Lack of financial resources to supplement needed food
- Lack of maternal bonding
- Substance abuse by the caretaker
- Significant or recent changes in the family makeup

Infants and toddlers with failure to thrive can appear emaciated, pale, have poor muscle tone, be listless, have periods of irritability, and may sleep for extended periods of time. Toddlers with severe failure to thrive may have a characteristic symptom known as *"frozen watchfulness"* (when they follow the movements of the people in the room with a look of fear). You may also see these children in a "frog like" position in the bed, with their arms and legs flexed. They may also exhibit rhythmic body movements such as head banging and body rocking. When assessing a child for failure to thrive you may see a decrease in height and weight followed by a decrease in head circumference. The head is the last of the measurements to decline in failure to thrive. If the head circumference is falling off the curve this is a very eminent sign.

Failure to thrive without the presence of an underlying disease process is usually related to difficulty in parenting. The cause is related to a lack of caloric intake, as well as the underlying problem with the parent child relationship or a lack of bonding.

Failure to thrive is a very serious form of child maltreatment when related to parental inadequacies. It must be aggressively identified and treated to prevent further harm to the child.

A comprehensive medical and social evaluation needs to be

completed to identify the cause.

Please refer to the four growth curve charts on the following pages. The authors gratefully acknowledge Ross Products Division, Abbott Laboratories for permission to include these charts in this text.

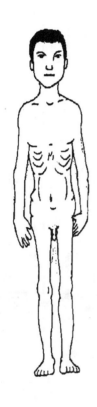

FAILURE TO THRIVE

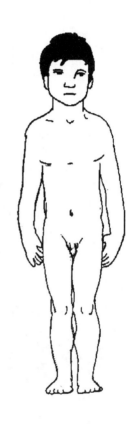

NORMAL

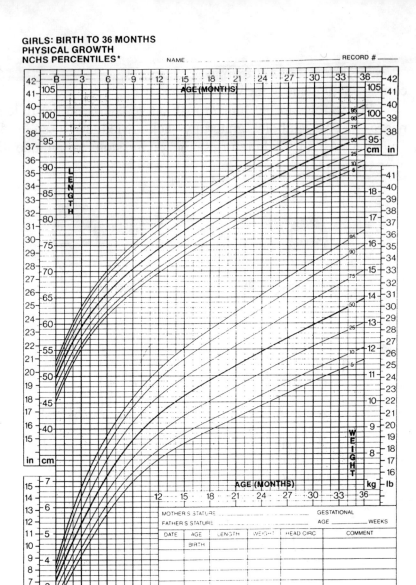

GIRLS: BIRTH TO 36 MONTHS
PHYSICAL GROWTH
NCHS PERCENTILES*

Adapted from: Hamill PVV, Drizd TA, Johnson CL, Reed RB, Roche AF, Moore WM: Physical growth: National Center for Health Statistics percentiles. AM J CLIN NUTR 32:607-629, 1979. Data from the Fels Longitudinal Study, Wright State University School of Medicine, Yellow Springs, Ohio.

Reprinted with permission of Ross Laboratories, Columbus, OH 43216. From NCHS Growth Charts, Copyright 1982 Ross Laboratories

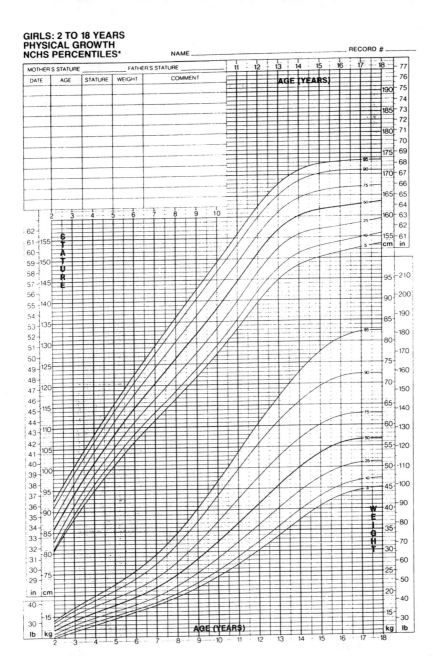

GIRLS: 2 TO 18 YEARS
PHYSICAL GROWTH
NCHS PERCENTILES*

Adapted from: Hamill PVV, Drizd TA, Johnson CL, Reed RB, Roche AF, Moore WM: Physical growth: National Center for Health Statistics percentiles. AM J CLIN NUTR 32:607-629, 1979. Data from the Fels Longitudinal Study, Wright State University School of Medicine, Yellow Springs, Ohio.

Reprinted with permission of Ross Laboratories, Columbus, OH 43216. From NCHS Growth Charts, Copyright 1982 Ross Laboratories

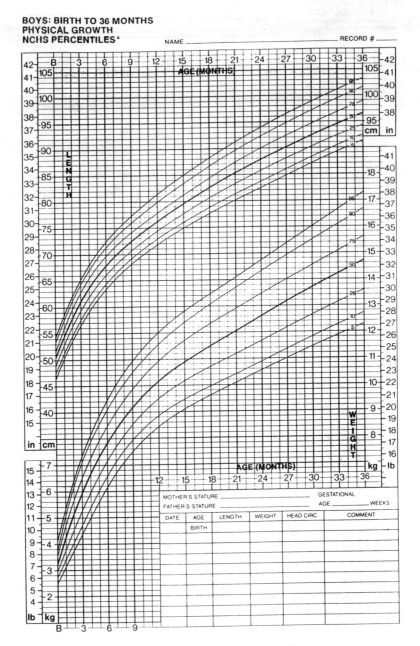

**BOYS: BIRTH TO 36 MONTHS
PHYSICAL GROWTH
NCHS PERCENTILES***

NAME _____ RECORD # _____

Adapted from: Hamill PVV, Drizd TA, Johnson CL, Reed RB, Roche AF, Moore WM: Physical growth: National Center for Health Statistics percentiles. AM J CLIN NUTR 32:607-629, 1979. Data from the National Center for Health Statistics (NCHS), Hyattsville, Maryland.

Reprinted with permission of Ross Laboratories, Columbus, OH 43216. From NCHS Growth Charts, Copyright 1982 Ross Laboratories

82

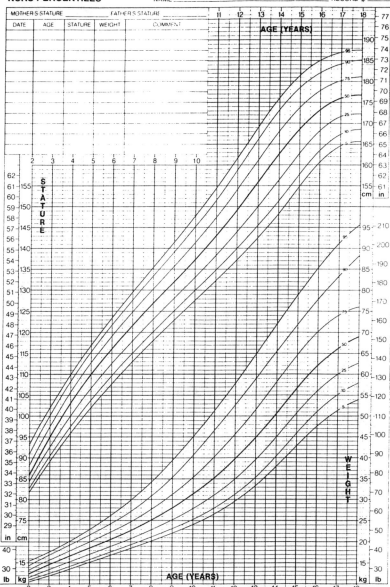

BOYS: 2 TO 18 YEARS
PHYSICAL GROWTH
NCHS PERCENTILES*

Adapted from: Hamill PVV, Drizd TA, Johnson CL, Reed RB, Roche AF, Moore WM: Physical growth: National Center for Health Statistics percentiles. AM J CLIN NUTR 32:607-629, 1979. Data from the National Center for Health Statistics (NCHS), Hyattsville, Maryland.

Reprinted with permission of Ross Laboratories, Columbus, OH 43216. From NCHS Growth Charts, Copyright 1982 Ross Laboratories

83

Protect Against Child Abuse

Think Abuse

1. *Poor physical growth*

2. *Delayed motor, social and cognitive development*

3. *Lack of maternal bonding*

4. *Substance abuse by the caregiver*

5. *Lack of appropriate medical management due to poor compliance*

CHAPTER TWELVE

MUNCHAUSEN SYNDROME BY PROXY

Munchausen Syndrome (also known as Fictitious Disorder) is a behavior where *a person fabricates symptoms or illnesses to gain medical attention.*

Munchausen Syndrome by Proxy (MSBP) is when the fabrication of medical symptoms and illnesses are perpetrated on another person such as a child. These behaviors when perpetrated on a child can produce injuries or life threatening consequences. (For the purposes of this book we will discuss the behaviors of the mother and the effects on the child).

MSBP is a psychological disorder that is defined in the *Diagnostic Statistic Manual of Mental Illness* (DSM IV). It is most commonly a disorder of women or female caretakers many of whom are pathological liars or have a personality disorder. The fabrication of the child's illness can often be related to the mother's feeling of being sick or in need of help. The female caretaker usually has knowledge of the medical community through a history of working in a medical setting, such as a nurse, physician, lab technician or nurses aide. The male caretaker is usually passive, not involved due to long working hours. He may not realize nor address the female caretakers behaviors. The female caretakers *behavior* is often *characterized* by:

⇨ Concern for their child

⇨ Eagerness to assist medical professionals

⇨ Knowledgeable about medical procedures

⇨ Knowledgeable of medical terms

⇨ Encourages further testing

⇨ Very attentive toward the child

⇨ Appears emotionally attached to the child

The *behavior* which causes the intentional harm to the child includes, but not limited to:

⇨ Interfering with diagnostic procedures

⇨ Turning the IV off causing the child to be repeatedly stuck by a needle

⇨ Administering ipecac to induce vomiting so that the child has a tangible symptom of illness

⇨ Giving the child mineral oil or ex-lax to cause diarrhea

⇨ Applying caustic chemicals to the skin to cause skin damage appearing as a diaper rash

⇨ Injecting bacteria into the IV causing serious infections

⇨ Exposing the child deliberately to harsh environmental substances such as cigarette smoke and or perfume causing the child to have breathing difficulty

⇨ In a child on anticonvulsants to prevent seizures, the caregiver will withhold the medication causing the continued seizure activity

⇨ Purposely suffocating the child with a pillow or plastic wrap causing the child to stop breathing which requires CPR measures and emergency care but not necessarily causing death.

Often these caregivers will utilize numerous emergency rooms, hospitals and physicians seeking medical care for fictitious illnesses. They will fabricate the medical history of previous hospitalizations and falsify diagnoses, medications and procedures the child has experienced. They will often claim that the previous physician was unable to provide the needed care for the child thus causing them to seek additional care. Often these care givers will progress through the medical system seeking more advanced medical centers and specialists. As the level and intensity of care increases the caregiver becomes more suspect by the practitioners in the advanced medical centers.

EXAMPLE OF CASE PRESENTATION

A common case presentation of a MSBP would be that of a "middle class, stay-at-home mom who previously worked as a lab technician in the local community hospital." Her husband is a traveling salesman, taking him away from home for long periods of time. There is a history of having multiple calls to 911(6 in 4 months). When the EMS arrive the mother is administering CPR to an unconscious, non- breathing child. All emergency episodes are characterized by the mother being alone with the child and no other witnesses present at the time of the incident. Extensive testing and evaluations yield no diagnostic results of illness. Her two year old child is a victim of MSBP.

MSBP can effect more than one or all of the children of the family. There is a high rate of child death related to this form of child abuse. The child's death is usually caused by the mother suffocating the child to death, or administrating a lethal overdose of poison or medication.

MSBP can be multigenerational or as a learned behavior of a child that can perpetuate in adult life.

Protect Against Child Abuse

THINK ABUSE

1. *Recurrent illnesses with no diagnosis*

2. *Inconsistencies between history and clinical findings*

3. *Unable to cure or make the child well*

4. *Closeness and fondness with the staff by mother*

5. *Allowing and encouraging multiple invasive procedures with no concern for the child's discomfort*

6. *Multiple hospitalization and evaluations with no resulting diagnosis*

Conclusion

*"The authors of this book provide us with an arsenal of knowledge to **fight the war on child abuse**. It's a must read for anyone who is compassionate to the needs of 'our' children."*

Maryann Russomano
Foster Parent

This book has given you the basic tools needed to identify and recognize child abuse. We hope that between these pages you are able to grasp the very difficult concept, that caretakers can seriously harm the children in their care.

We hope that this information provides you with the confidence to identify and report child abuse.

To fight the war against child abuse it is necessary to have an arsenal of information and tools to work with.

The war against child abuse begins with you.

RESOURCES

American Academy of Pediatrics
Publications Department
PO Box 927
141 Northwest Point Blvd.
Elk Grove Village, IL 60009-0927
(800) 433-9016

American Humane Association, Children's Division
63 Inverness Drive East
Englewood, CO 80112-5117
(303) 792-9900

Boys Town
Communications and Public Service Division
Father Flanagan's Boys' Home
Boys Town, NE 68101
(402) 498-1111   Hotline: (800) 448-3000

Children's Defense Fund
122 'C' Street, NW, Suite 400
Washington, DC 20001
(202) 628-8787

Children's Welfare League of America
440 First Street, NW, Suite 310
Washington, DC 20402-9325
(202) 638-2952

Resources

Family Help Line: 1-800-THE KIDS

Kempe Center Programs
Henry Kempe National Center for the Prevention and Treatment
of Child Abuse and Neglect
University of Colorado Health Sciences Center Department o
Pediatrics
1205 Oneida Street
Denver, CO 80220
303 321 3963

National Center for Education in Maternal & Child Health
38th and 'R' Streets, NW
Washington, DC 20057
(202) 625-8400

National Clearinghouse on Child Abuse and Neglect Information
PO Box 1182
Washington, DC 20013-1182
(800) FYI-3366
Fax: (703) 385-3206

New Jersey Department of Human Services
Division of Youth and Family Services
(800) 792-8610

Resources

Pediatric Projects
PO Box 1880
Santa Monica, CA 90406
(213) 828-8963

"Plain Talk" and *"Caring About Kids"* Series
US Department of Health and Human Services
Public Health Service
Alcohol, Drug Abuse, and Mental Health Association
5600 Fishers Lane
Rockville, MD 20857
(301) 443-3875

REFERENCES

Alexander, R.; Smith, W., and Stevenson, R. (1990). *Serial munchausen syndrome by proxy. Pediatrics.* 86(4).

American Academy of Pediatrics, Committee on Child Abuse and Neglect. (1993). *Shaken baby syndrome: Inflicted cerebral trauma. Pediatrics.* 92(6). 98-101.

American Academy of Pediatrics (1996). *Focus on child abuse: Resources for prevention, recognition and treatment.* (CD ROM). CMC Medical Division.

American Psychiatric Association. (1994). *Diagnostic and statistical manual of mental disorders* (4th Ed). Washington, DC. American Psychiatric Association.

Bates, B. (1983). *A guide to physical examination* (3rd Ed). Philadelphia. J.B. Lippincott.

Besharov, D.J. (1990). *Recognizing child abuse.* New York. The Free Press.

Black, M.M.; Dubowitz, H., Hutcheson, J., Berenson-Howard, J., and Starr, R.H. (1995). *A randomized clinical trial of home intervention for children with failure to thrive. Pediatrics.* 95(6). 807-814.

Dubowitz, H., and Jenny, C. (Eds.). (1997). *Child Maltreatment. Journal of the American Professional Society on the Abuse of Children.* 2(4).

Eberlein, T. (1997). *A moment's rage, a baby's life. Women's Day.* 120-123.

Finkelhor, D. (1986) *A sourcebook on child sexual abuse.* Thousand Oaks. Sage Publications, Inc.

REFERENCES

Hamilton, B.S. (1994) *The hidden legacy: Uncovering, confronting and healing three generations of incest*. Cypress House.

Helfer, RE. and Kempe, RS. (1988). *The battered child.* Chicago. The University of Chicago Press.

Huff, T.G. (1997). *Killing children by fire: Filicide: A preliminary analysis. The National Child Advocate*. 1(1). 4-5.

Jones. D.P.H. (1992). *Interviewing the sexually abused child: Investigation of suspected abuse*. Colorado. Gaskell.

Justice, B. and Justice, R. (1990). *The abusing family.* New York. Insight Books.

McGuire, E.V. (1997). *An under utilized resource. Update.* National Center for Protection of Child Abuse. 10(4/5).

Meadow, R. (1992). *Munchausen syndrome by proxy. Archives of Disease in Childhood*. (57), 92-98.

Mitchell, I., Brummitt, J., DeForest, J., and Fisher, G. (1993). *Apnea and factitious Illness (munchausen syndrome) by proxy. Pediatrics*. 92(6).

Monteleone, J.A. and Brodeur, A.E. (1994). *Child maltreatment: A clinical guide and reference*. St. Louis. G.W. Medical Publishing.

Monteleone, J.A. (1994). *Child Maltreatment: A comprehensive photographic reference identifying potential child abuse*. St. Louis. G.W. Medical Publishing.

Taylor, L. and Mauer, A. (1993). *Think twice: The medical effects of physical punishment*. Berkely. Generation Books.

Toufexis, A. (1994). *When is crib death a cover for murder? Time*. 63-64.

REFERENCES

Tower, C.C. (1996). *Understanding child abuse and neglect.* Portland. Allyn & Bacon.

Walters, S.B. (1996). *Principles of kinesic interview and interrogation.* Boca Raton. CRC Press.

INDEX

Abuse
  emotional 10,18
    indicators 15
    behavioral 18, 19
      of caretaker 19
      of victim 18
    physical 18
      of victim 18
  indicators 15
    behavioral 17
      of caretaker 17
      of victim 16
    physical 16
      of victim 16
  interviewing 8, 11
    establishing the setting 11
    general rules 13
    interviewer 12
  legal liability 11
  neglect 22
    indicators 22, 23
    behavioral 22
      of caretaker 23
      of victim 22
    physical 22
      of victim 22
  reporting 8
    obligations/legal considerations 8
    risk of harm 8
  sexual 19
    indicators 19
    behavioral 20
      of caretaker 20
      of victim 20
    physical 19
      of victim 19

Assessment
  Physical 24
    normal child 24, 27, 28, 29
  psychosocial 1

Burns 60
  contact 62, 63, 64
  filicide 67
  immersion 66
  scalding 65

Injuries
  abdominal 68
  chest 68
  genital 72
    vaginal 74
    penile 75
  factures 30
    comminuted 34
    compound/open 33
    epiphyseal-metaphyseal 36
    impacted 37
    linear 39
    rib 38
    simple/closed 32
    skull 39
      depressed 39, 40
    spiral/oblique 30, 31
    transverse 35
  head 42
    hematoma 44
    hemorrages 44
      epidural 45
      retinal 45
      subdural 44
      subgaleal 45
      traumatic alopecia 45
    shaken baby syndrome 42, 43
  skin 47
    locations 48
      back/chest/abdominal 51
      buttocks 52
      ear 49
      eye 50
      mouth 49
    types
      abrasion 47
      bruise 47, 53

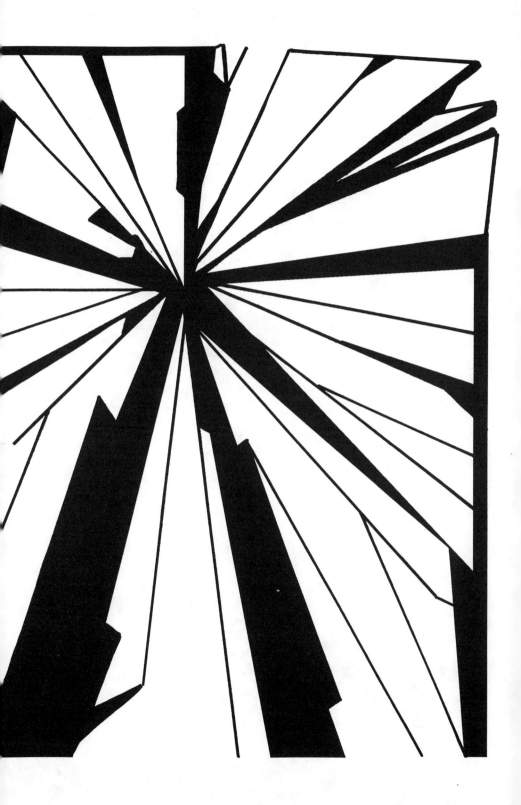

ATTENTION NURSES!!